Student Workbook to Accompany

Contemporary Medical Office Procedures

Third Edition

Doris D. Humphrey, Ph.D.
President, Career Solutions Training Group

THOMSON
DELMAR LEARNING™

Australia Canada Mexico Singapore Spain United Kingdom United States

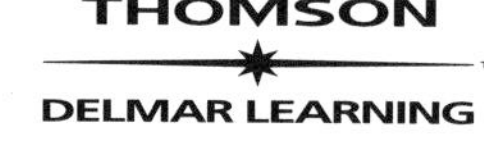

Student Workbook to Accompany Contemporary Medical Office Procedures, Third Edition
by Doris D. Humphrey, PhD

Vice President, Health Care SBU:
William Brottmiller

Editorial Director:
Cathy L. Esperti

Acquisitions Editor:
Rhonda Dearborn

Editorial Assistant:
Natalie Wager

Developmental Editor:
Mary Ellen Cox

Marketing Director:
Jennifer McAvey

Channel Manager:
Lisa Osgood

Marketing Coordinator:
Mona Caron

Technology Specialist:
Victoria Moore

Production Coordinator:
Jessica Peterson

Project Editor:
Bryan Viggiani

Art and Design Coordinator:
Connie Lundberg-Watkins

Printed in the United States of America
4 5 6 GP 08 07 06

For more information contact Delmar Learning, 5 Maxwell Drive, Clifton Park, NY 12065

Or find us on the World Wide Web at http://www.delmarlearning.com

Library of Congress Catalog No. 2003055064

ISBN 1-4018-7068-6

NOTICE TO THE READER

Publisher does not warrant or guarantee any of the products described herein or perform any independent analysis in connection with any of the product information contained herein. Publisher does not assume, and expressly disclaims, any obligation to obtain and include information other than that provided to it by the manufacturer.

The reader is expressly warned to consider and adopt all safety precautions that might be indicated by the activities described herein and to avoid all potential hazards. By following the instructions contained herein, the reader willingly assumes all risks in connection with such instructions.

The publisher makes no representations or warranties of any kind, including but not limited to, the warranties of fitness for particular purpose or merchantability, nor are any such representations implied with respect to the material set forth herein, and the publisher takes no responsibility with respect to such material. The publisher shall not be liable for any special, consequential, or exemplary damages resulting, in whole or part, from the reader's use of, or reliance upon, this material.

Table of Contents

Preface

As the physician's job has become more complex under managed care, the medical assistant's responsibilities have broadened. Medical assistants are expected to apply knowledge in many areas, ranging from understanding the highly legislated managed care community to interacting with patients and coordinating the daily schedule, to using sophisticated technology for communication and record keeping, to demonstrating in-depth critical thinking and problem-solving skills. The dynamic, often rushed, atmosphere of a medical setting requires each medical assistant to demonstrate an excellent attitude—one that translates into cooperation, acceptance of responsibility, and the desire to continue learning.

This *Student Workbook to Accompany Contemporary Medical Office Procedures,* Third Edition, was written to help the learner review concepts presented in the textbook and to assist students in gaining the knowledge and skills needed to be successful. It encourages the application of medical office assisting knowledge in a variety of learning situations. It may be used with the *Contemporary Medical Office Procedures* textbook or as a text-workbook for short segments of learning or individualized study. This student workbook can be incorporated into many classes with varying time schedules.

Suggestions for Using the Student Workbook

Each chapter of the workbook extends the material contained in the matching chapters of the textbook. Look for these components:

- Key Vocabulary Terms test the students' knowledge of the chapter vocabulary.
- Chapter Review questions assess the students' understanding of the chapter content.
- Critical Thinking Scenarios challenge the students to assume the role of a medical office assistant and make decisions.
- "Day-in-the-Life" Simulations require students to perform real-life tasks that they might encounter in a medical practice.
- The workbook is correlated to Delmar's Medical Assisting CD-ROM. Most chapters of the workbook direct students to the CD-ROM to complete an activity.
- The instructor's manual for *Contemporary Medical Office Procedures,* Third Edition, includes a special section devoted to the workbook. In this section, you will find solutions to all chapter activities and recommended answers to the Day-in-the-Life simulations.

Key Vocabulary Terms

Match each word or term with its correct meaning.

____	1. On call		a. concentration on specific body systems
____	2. CDC		b. full bill paid each time a patient visits the physician
____	3. Third-party reimbursement		c. physicians and hospitals compete for patients
____	4. Fee-for-service		d. three years of specialty training
____	5. Managed competition		e. basic medical word plus prefix or suffix
____	6. Medical specialties		f. availability on an as-needed basis
____	7. Residency		g. someone other than the patient pays
____	8. Root medical word		h. Atlanta research center

Chapter Review

1. Why are health care costs rising in the United States?

2. How have high costs of medical care changed the physician's work?

3. How have the high costs of medical care affected the medical assistant's work?

4. How do the rising costs of medical malpractice insurance affect society?

5. What factors are contributing to the increase in jobs available for medical assistants?

6. Why is documentation of medical records more important today than ever before?

7. Why are group practices becoming more common among doctors?

8. In what ways has the Centers for Medicare & Medicaid Services affected medical assistants?

9. What importance has the Health Insurance Portability Act had on health care reform?

____

____

____

____

10. Computers are used in medicine for many administrative and diagnostic purposes. For each of the following, write an *A* to identify the purpose as *Administrative* and a *D* to identify the purpose as *Diagnostic*.

    ____ Analyze and refine patient data from laboratory tests

    ____ Maintain a record of a patient's health

    ____ Suggest an illness after test results are entered

    ____ Cross-check drugs

    ____ Show magnetic resonance imaging scans

    ____ Store and access a physician's instructions to nurses

    ____ Maintain a database of correct dosages based on patient weight

    ____ Send a picture of a patient's heart from a remote location to a large hospital

    ____ Analyze and interpret information about a diseased body part

Critical Thinking Scenarios

1. Wicha Rafer soon will be graduating from a two-year medical assisting program. Recently, she had the following conversation with a friend. Assume you are the friend. What advice will you give Wicha?

   "I just can't decide whether to work in a solo practice or a group practice. The idea of working in a big practice with several doctors is exciting, but it's also appealing to think that in a solo practice I would work closely with one doctor. I don't think I have any other choices though. What's your advice?"

____

____

____

____

____

____

2. After sending out resumes for six weeks, your neighbor, Joel Reddy, has been called to interview for a medical assistant position at two practices. One practice contracts with an EPO, and the other is part of an HMO that offers a Point-of-Service Plan. Joel calls you in a panic the night before the first interview and says, "I still get confused about what all these acronyms mean. Tell me again what the difference is between an EPO and a POS Plan."

3. During your internship rotation as a medical assistant, you had an opportunity to work in three different specialties or subspecialties: a dermatology practice, a family practice, and an emergency medicine practice. A student who is just entering the medical assisting program asks you to describe what each practice does and the type of patients it sees. What will you tell her?

4. As program director for your local AAMA chapter, you have invited a panel of dental specialists to discuss job opportunities in their field. To start the program, you will introduce the dentists, then give a short summary of the dental specialties of the American Dental Association. You have two minutes for your part of the program.

5. The young endocrinologist for whom you work is thinking about developing a research project using his patients as subjects. He is interested in many different disorders and illnesses, so he is open to researching in a variety of areas. He believes that he can secure funding for the research from either the Centers for Disease Control and Prevention or the National Institutes of Health. Because of his busy schedule, he asks you to research the Internet for available grants, then to summarize for him the work these two leading institutions are doing. Use the following Web sites for your research: http://www.cdc.gov and http://www.nih.gov.

6. You have been invited back to the school where you received your medical assisting training to speak to a class of entering medical assistants. The new students are very focused. Within weeks of the start of school, many already have decided what area of medicine interests them most as a field of work; however, some have not yet connected their interests with the body systems. Tell Clarissa, Alan, Maria, Pia, Juan, Anna, Ling, and Sean the body system that relates most closely to their interests.

_______________ Clarissa is a former gymnast. She would like to combine her interest in medicine with body movement.

_______________ As a child, Alan's bloody cuts and scrapes were fascinating because they usually healed without help from a doctor. When he was older, he routinely volunteered to donate blood and volunteered at the Red Cross. The role of blood to body functioning intrigues him.

_______________ Maria loves babies, and stories about difficult pregnancies, premature births, problem deliveries, and infertility capture her interest.

_______________ Pia is a brain; everyone says so. Therefore, it is no surprise that she is interested in how the brain tells the body what to do and how to do it.

_______________ Juan's mom was sick until she was diagnosed with hyperthyroidism and swallowed radioactive iodine to eliminate her thyroid gland. Since then, Juan has been amazed at her progress. He would like to work in a field that helps him learn more about this and similar illnesses.

_______________ Anna's animals were easy to identify in her neighborhood as she was growing up, for their legs were usually in a cast. At one point, she adopted a three-legged pug who ended up with a peg leg of her design. It is a foregone conclusion that she wants to work with broken bones.

_______________ After Ling's grandma died of lung cancer and his uncle was sick for years with emphysema, there was never a question that he would work with a doctor who treats these illnesses.

_______________ Sean was an EMT in high school and saw many burn victims whose lost large portions of their skin in fires. He has witnessed the terrible suffering and the miraculous healing that can occur when the skin is involved, and he is determined to learn more.

circulatory system	the heart, blood vessels, blood, and lymphatic system
digestive system	organs and glands associated with ingestion and digestion of food
endocrine system	glands that regulate body functions, including the adrenal, pituitary, thyroid, and sex glands
integumentary system	nails, hair, skin and related appendages
muscular system	more than 600 muscles that contract and pull tissue to create body movement
nervous system	brain, spinal cord, and others that regulate and coordinate the activities of all the other systems
respiratory system	organs that allow breathing
reproductive system	organs that enable men and women to have children
skeletal system	bones that support and protect the body
urinary system	filters wastes from the blood and flushes them from the body through urine

Simulations Introduction

The simulations you are about to begin represent the work you will perform during your first fifteen days at Graupera and Marks—one simulation for each day. After completing all fifteen simulations, one referenced to each chapter of the textbook, you will have experienced most of the activities typically performed by a medical assistant in any private practice. Save all the Action Papers in each simulation because you will need them later.

Simulation Scenario

Your First Job

Congratulations! You have just been hired by Dr. Judith Marks and Dr. Ramon Graupera, specialists in internal medicine and cardiology at Marks and Graupera, P.C., 2201 Locust Street, Philadelphia, PA 19101. Telephone: 215-283-8372; fax: 215-283-2938; e-mail: MG@MarksandGraupera.com. You are on your way to an exciting career in Philadelphia, Pennsylvania.

Medical assisting positions with Dr. Marks, the senior physician and cardiologist, and Dr. Graupera, the managing physician and internal medical specialist, are coveted because the doctors expect a great deal from their staff and reward them with interesting challenges and excellent pay. They provide all new medical assistants with three weeks of intensive training that is thorough, challenging, and enjoyable. Working with these well-respected physicians is prestigious and forms the foundation for a rewarding career.

You will work with other staff members. Suzanne Romez, a physician's assistant, and Luke Streeter, a clinical medical assistant, report to Dr. Marks. Lydia Makay, CMA, office manager; Tarik Loper, clinical administrative assistant; and you, report to Dr. Graupera.

Dr. Marks is a 1965 graduate of the University of Pennsylvania School of Medicine and Dr. Graupera is a 1963 graduate of Vanderbilt University School of Medicine. Dr. Marks's Social Security number is 415-55-4321 and Dr. Graupera's Social Security number is 365-55-1061.

Marks and Graupera is located in downtown Philadelphia, near Independence Hall, the Liberty Bell, and the Constitution Center. Benjamin Franklin is buried nearby and George Washington led the Battle of Valley Forge a few miles away. The Hospital of the University of Pennsylvania, Pennsylvania Children's Hospital, and Jefferson Hospital are a short walk or taxi ride away. You are lucky in many ways; you will be working for great doctors and walking on the same streets as the signers of the Declaration of Independence and will be near some of America's most prestigious medical research and treatment centers.

Good luck in your new position.

Simulation Preparation

1. Prepare fifteen file folders with labels—one file folder for each of fifteen simulations. Label each folder with the simulation number and your name (Simulation 1: First name and last name).
2. Before starting a simulation, review the chapter in the textbook that the simulation matches. For example, Chapter 1 should be reviewed before beginning Simulation 1.

Simulation Procedures

1. Organize the Action Papers for the simulation in numerical order. Keep all papers for the simulation together. Read each of the papers, including all handwritten instructions.
2. Rate the urgency of each task using the categories below:

   Rush—Tasks on which action should be taken immediately

   ASAP—Tasks on which action should be taken as soon as all Rush items are completed

   Routine—Tasks that can be carried over to another day, if necessary
3. Mark the urgency of each Action Paper in Section 1 of the Work Summary (found at the end of the chapter). To do this, list each Action Paper number (shown in the upper right corner of the Action Paper) in its correct category: Rush, ASAP, or Routine. Your instructor will use the Work Summary for evaluation purposes.
4. Complete a To Do List with a brief description of each action to be taken. You will find a blank To Do List following the Action Papers.

5. Read the Supplies Needed and the Action Options, Suggestions, and Conflicts sections that come right before the Action Papers begin. Gather the supplies you will need (many are included in your workbook, but there are some things you will need to supply, such as blank paper), then perform the tasks indicated by each Action Paper. Some tasks will include instructions, whereas the proper handling of others will be left for you to decide on. Because your time each day in the medical office is limited, and patients generate a great deal of work, use the most efficient processes and procedures to complete each task.
6. Check off each task on your To Do List as it is completed.
7. Place each Action Paper in its simulation folder. Clip to it any accompanying papers you generate.
8. Follow the same procedure with the next simulation.
9. Merge leftover work from a previous day with the next day's papers and reprioritize as needed.

Simulation 1

Supplies Needed

Reply e-mail form
Blank note form
Blank paper
To Do List
Work Summary

Action Options, Suggestions, and Conflicts

- Use the blank e-mail forms that are provided if you do not have access to e-mail, or key and print e-mail messages directly from the computer if you have access to e-mail.
- Telephone conversations are identified by an illustration of a telephone at the top of an Action Paper.
- Face-to-face conversations are identified by an illustration of people at the top of an Action Paper.
- When reference is made to a CD-ROM, use the CD-ROM that accompanies your textbook. These activities are identified by an illustration of a CD at the top of an Action Paper.
- If a form becomes too messy to use because of corrections or other reasons, obtain and copy a blank form from your instructor or use plain paper. Label the form appropriately.

Name: ______________________ Date: ______________

Action Paper 1-1

Please complete the chart so you'll have a clear idea of the reporting order.
Lydia

Organization Chart

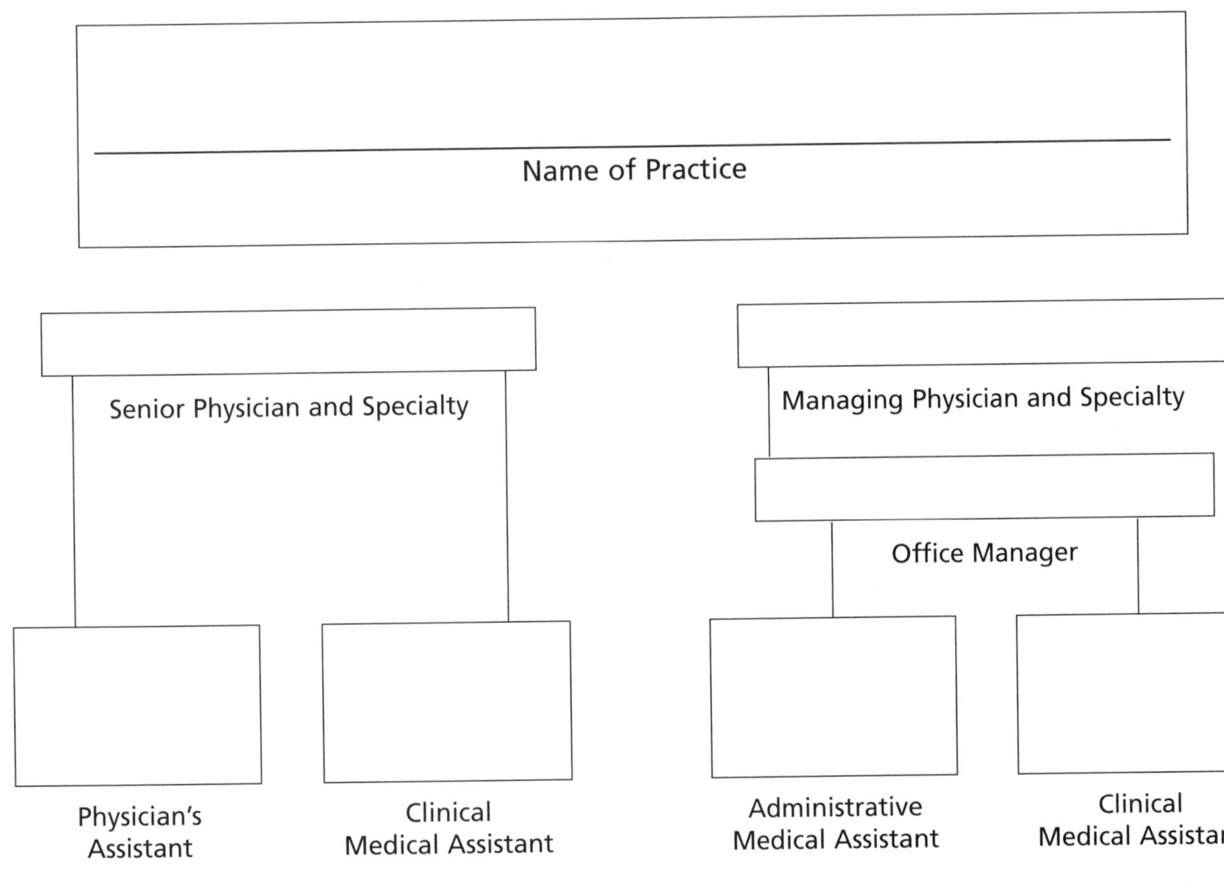

Name: ______________________ Date: ______________

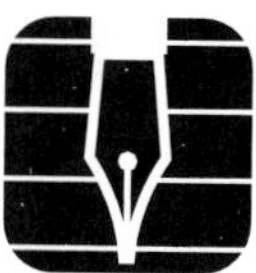

Action Paper 1-2

To: Your name@MarksandGraupera.com
From: TarikLoper@MarksandGraupera.com
Subject: Lunch

Hi, you've been in meetings with Lydia all morning, so I haven't had a chance to say much more than hello. Would you like to go to lunch? I'll fill you in on some of the things you'll need to know.

I'm glad you came to work here. You'll like it. Dr. Graupera is great. So is Dr. Marks, but you won't see as much of her.

E-mail me back about lunch.

Reply To: TarikLoper@MarksandGraupera.com
From: Your name@MarksandGraupera.com
Subject: Lunch

Name: ______________________________ Date: ______________

Action Paper 1-3

Dr. Graupera: "I just finished a brief examination of Maryellen Reynolds, who is still in the examining room. Write Tarik a note to schedule her for a complete physical exam and an electrocardiogram, then to send her to the lab for a complete blood count, a thyroid profile, and a urinalysis. Tell him to give her written instructions of the medications: Tylenol as needed and at bedtime. By the way, use medical abbreviations in your note to Tarik. That's what he is used to seeing."

You: "All right, I will."

Name: ____________________ Date: ____________

Action Paper 1-4

Tarik: "A few years ago we made up a glossary of the words and terms that our practice uses frequently. It has been very helpful to me, and we've recorded it on CD for new medical assistants. Here's my copy of the CD. Why don't you look at the terms and start a notebook of any definitions you aren't familiar with, in case the docs use a term you don't know."

You: "Thanks."

Name: ______________________ Date: ______________

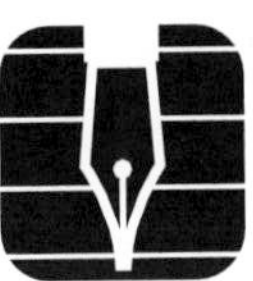

Action Paper 1-5

Marks and Graupera, P.C.

Note from Lydia

Sorry I had to run out on you. The accountant called, and I had to spend some time with him. How about us continuing our meeting at lunch? There's a good place nearby where we can have a sandwich and finish up the details that will help you get started. I'll be busy tomorrow so we won't have a chance to spend too much time together. Write a note on this sheet and leave it on my desk telling me what time you prefer to go. I'm flexible.

Lydia

Name: ______________________ Date: ______________

To Do List

-
-
-
-
-
-
-
-
-
-
-
-
-
-
-
-
-

Name: ______________________

Date Started: ______________ Date Completed: ______________

Work Summary 1

Section 1

1. Record the numbers of the Action Papers marked "Rush." ________
2. Record the numbers of the Action Papers marked "ASAP." ________
3. Record the numbers of the Action Papers marked "Routine." ________

Section 2

4. Write the list of "To Do" items and the actions that were taken. When this section is complete, turn the Work Summary over to your instructor, who will evaluate your work and return it for your later use.

To Do	Action Taken

Section 3

5. You will receive two assessments for your work—one is based on time to complete the items and the other is based on quality of work. Your instructor will complete the Assessment portion of the Work Summary.

			Points Received
Time Required			________
	20 points	25 minutes or less	
	15 points	30 minutes	
	10 points	35 minutes	
	5 points	40 minutes	
Quality of Work			________
		Total Points	________

Name: ______________________ Date: ______________

CHAPTER 2
The Medical Staff

Chapter Outline

- The Medical Assistant
  - Certification
  - Career Opportunities
  - The Multiskilled Medical Assistant
  - Responsibilities of the Position
  - The Role Delineation Study Analysis
  - Job Titles and Job Sites
- The Roles of Medical Professionals
  - Physicians
  - Physician Extenders
  - Nurses
  - Medical Technologists and Technicians
  - Medical Records Personnel
- Working with the Medical Professionals
  - Working with the Physician and the Health Care Team
    - Honesty
    - Cooperation
    - Assertiveness
    - Dependability
    - Loyalty
  - Coordinating with the Hospital Staff
  - Interacting with Other Outside Professionals
- Chapter Activities
  - Performance-Based Activities
  - Expanding Your Thinking

Key Vocabulary Terms

Match each word or term with its correct meaning.

_____	1. Ambulatory care centers	a. trained support staff for physician
_____	2. CMA	b. Role Delineation Chart
_____	3. CPT	c. administrative and clinical training
_____	4. Credentialing	d. twenty-four-hour medical centers
_____	5. Multiskilled medical assistant	e. medical assistant accrediting group
_____	6. OMA	f. Current Procedural Terminology
_____	7. Physician extenders	g. medical assistant organization
_____	8. RMA	h. Certified Medical Assistant
_____	9. AAMA	i. examination for office procedures
_____	10. CAAHEP	j. Registered Medical Assistant
_____	11. RDC	k. Ophthalmic Medical Assistant

Chapter Review

1. Name several specific job titles, such as receptionist, that fall under the broad category of medical assistant.

2. How does an administrative medical assistant's work differ from the work of a clinical medical assistant and a multiskilled medical assistant?

3. What is required to become a Certified Medical Assistant?

4. Name several responsibilities of an administrative medical assistant.

5. Name several responsibilities of a clinical medical assistant.

6. Why is the Role Delineation Chart important?

____

____

____

____

7. What suppport does a medical assistant provide to a physician?

____

____

____

____

8. Identify several tasks of a support nature that medical assistants perform to help other medical professionals in the office.

____

____

____

____

9. Why is the medical assistant job category growing in number of positions?

____

____

____

____

10. Why are job opportunities better for a certified medical assistant than for a noncertified medical assistant?

____

____

____

____

____

Critical Thinking Scenarios

1. After graduating from a medical assisting program, you decide to expand your knowledge of the United States by starting your career in another city. After researching the Internet, you discover the number of medical assisting positions that are projected to be available this year in six cities. Because you are not sure whether you prefer to work in a primary care, surgical, or other specialty, you use the percentages published by the AAMA to calculate approximately how many positions might be available in each specialty in each city. Based on the information in the AAMA chart on page 21 of the textbook, calculate and list the numbers in each position in each city.

   City No. 1 219 positions total

   __________ primary care __________ surgical __________ other

   City No. 2 529 positions total

   __________ primary care __________ surgical __________ other

   City No. 3 370 positions total

   __________ primary care __________ surgical __________ other

   City No. 4 134 positions total

   __________ primary care __________ surgical __________ other

   City No. 5 77 positions total

   __________ primary care __________ surgical __________ other

   City No. 6 402 positions total

   __________ primary care __________ surgical __________ other

2. Tuan, Rebecca, and Judy have applied at the dermatology practice where you work as an office manager. From their descriptions, which person do you think should specialize in **administrative tasks**, which should specialize in **clinical tasks**, and which should pursue a job that involves **multiple skills**.

   __________ Tuan likes to work alone where he can concentrate on a task or a puzzling problem. Though he enjoys being around people occasionally, he often becomes tired and irritable when he is surrounded by others. Tuan is great with details, and you can trust any work he does to be complete and accurate.

   __________ Rebecca has been juggling projects as long as she can remember. She is active in many different groups and often is appointed as the group's leader because she can be depended on to follow through until a project is completed. She likes to know how to do many different things, and she works hard to be good at what she does. In fact, Rebecca gets bored if she has to concentrate on one thing for too long.

   __________ Judy puts people at ease in difficult situations. She gains their confidence and is able to help them overcome their insecurities. She is one of those people you can trust to make you feel better because her personality is warm and caring. Judy is surprised that she is known as a "people person" because her real love is science and physiology, a field that is more focused on facts and statistics.

3. Ratha starts next week as a medical assistant in the pediatric practice where you work. Several individuals with different titles work at Pediatric Partners, P.C., and Ratha wants to become as knowledgeable as possible about their responsibilities before her first day. She asks you to tell her what each staff member does. Later, she will determine in what way she will be working with each.

   Dr. Romez, pediatrician

   ____

   ____

   ____

   ____

   Anita, physician assistant

   ____

   ____

   ____

   ____

   Gordon, medical technologist

   ____

   ____

   ____

   ____

   Sung-Li, medical records technician

   ____

   ____

   ____

   ____

4. As senior medical assistant at Chairson and Lopez, P.C., you have been assigned to mentor Kathi Polenski, who came to work four weeks ago. Lately, you have made notes about Kathi's observable behaviors that concern you. Now it is time to talk to her. Kathi has strong opinions and says what she thinks. One staff member has called Kathi "pushy" and says she is uncooperative. As you have watched the situation unfold, you have come to believe that Kathi is like many new graduates who need to aggressively establish how smart they are because they think they gain respect. What will you say?

   ____

   ____

   ____

   ____

5. As a medical assistant at Devon Medical Center, you have learned that working with other staff is often a challenge. Sometimes it is hard to know the right thing to do. A conversation you had with another medical assistant this morning (shown below) is disturbing, and you are trying to decide how you should have handled it. What should you have done?

   Duana: "Dr. Bolling's schedule for tomorrow morning shows she's out until 10:00 on a personal appointment. Don't tell anyone I said this, but I think she's pregnant and trying to hide it. I saw her coming out of the OB/GYN's office on the third floor when I took the elevator yesterday. Since she's going to be late, I'm going to sneak in late, too. Cover for me, and she'll never know. I shouldn't be more than thirty minutes late."

   ____

   ____

   ____

   ____

6. Duana, identified above, guessed wrong. Dr. Bolling arrived on time this morning, as did a patient she had consulted with on the phone last night and had asked to come in early. You are busy with a patient of Dr. Janeway's and can offer minimum assistance. Dr. Bolling appears irritated and asks you why Duana is late.

   ____

   ____

   ____

   ____

7. You are attending a seminar on "Managing the Administrative Staff" after being promoted to office manager at Frazier Radiology Associates. As part of a small group discussion, you are asked to name and discuss the traits you think are most important in getting along with other staff, including the physicians.

   ____

   ____

   ____

   ____

8. Shyness is a trait you wish you could overcome. You do your job well; you are well respected and you feel comfortable with yourself most of the time. But you hate confrontation and often agree to things when you would prefer to disagree. At lunch, you are so frustrated that you complain about yourself to Elana, your friend. She says, "I know what I think, but you tell me what you can do to change."

   ____

   ____

   ____

   ____

Simulation 2

Today is your second day of work at Marks and Graupera. Review the Simulation Preparation and Procedures instructions from Simulation 1 and process today's papers in the same manner.

Supplies Needed

Role Delineation Chart
Blank paper
Notepaper
To Do List
Work Summary

Action Options, Suggestions, and Conflicts

Several things you need to think about as you make decisions today are listed below.

- At lunch today, you are planning to return a pair of pants that are too large.
- Lydia has scheduled you to spend the afternoon getting up-to-date on the computer system. She has asked you to plan to work with another employee from 1:00 to 5:00, the normal end of the day. Tonight you are meeting a friend at the gym at 5:30 to work out.

Name: ______________________ Date: ______________

Action Paper 2-1

Marks and Graupera, P.C.

Note from Dr. Marks

Sorry I was out of the office for your first day of work. We are pleased you have joined us. You had excellent references, and we're expecting great things from you. I would like to spend some time with you this afternoon. I am available at 1:30, 4:30, and 5:45. Please return this note telling me your preference.

Name: ____________________ Date: ____________

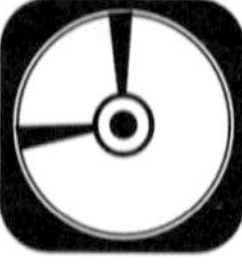

Action Paper 2-2

To: Your name@MarksandGraupera.com
From: TarikLoper@MarksandGraupera.com
Subject: Lunch

Do you still have my CD of the practice's glossary? Getting familiar with a few more terms with help you since we use them a lot. Why don't you add these to the notebook we talked about?

professional courtesy
nonverbal behavior
pharmaceutical representative
health maintenance organization
employee handbook

professional
medical assistant
oral communication skills
employee
partnership

Name: ____________________ Date: ____________

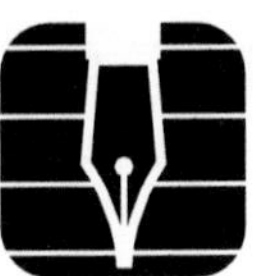

Action Paper 2-3

Marks and Graupera, P.C.

Note from Tarik

Since Lydia preempted me yesterday at lunch, let's try to go to lunch today. The office closes from 12:00 to 1:00 every day for lunch. Let me know.

T. L.

Name: ______________________ Date: ______________

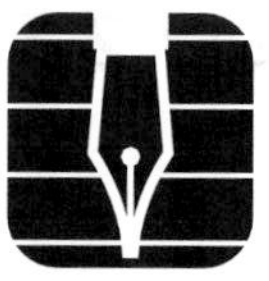

Action Paper 2-4

To: Your name@MarksandGraupera.com
From: LydiaMakay@MarksandGraupera.com
Subject: Task list

To get you off to a good start, Dr. Graupera and I would like to assign tasks that take advantage of your best skills and strengths. Will you please rate your skill level in each area on the attached chart as Basic, Above Average, or Excellent? Thanks.

Marks and Graupera Task List

Taken from the AAMA Role Delineation Chart

Administrative Procedures

_____ Perform basic clerical functions
_____ Perform basic administrative medical assisting functions
_____ Schedule, coordinate, and monitor appointments
_____ Schedule inpatient/outpatient admissions and procedures
_____ Understand and apply third-party guidelines
_____ Obtain reimbursement through accurate claims submission
_____ Monitor third-party reimbursement
_____ Understand and adhere to managed care policies and procedures
_____ *Negotiate managed care contracts

Practice Finance

_____ Perform procedural and diagnostic testing
_____ Apply bookkeeping principles
_____ Manage accounts receivable
_____ *Manage accounts payable
_____ *Process payroll
_____ *Document and maintain accounting and banking records
_____ *Document and maintain fee schedules
_____ *Manage renewals of business and professional insurance policies
_____ *Manage personnel benefits and maintain records
_____ *Perform marketing, financial, and strategic planning

*Denotes advanced skills.

Name: ______________________ Date: ______________

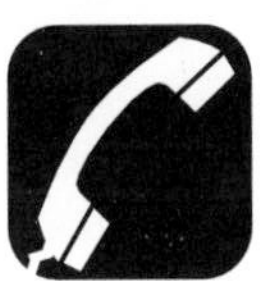

Action Paper 2-5

Caller: Hi, it's Janie, how is the new job?

You: I like it.

Caller: Remember when we talked a few weeks ago, and I said I was thinking about pursuing CMA certification? You seemed to know a lot about certification. I can't remember everything you said. When you have a chance, will you send me an e-mail of what I have to do to become certified?

You: Sure, as soon as I get a chance.

Name: ______________________ Date: ______________

To Do List

-
-
-
-
-
-
-
-
-
-
-
-
-
-
-
-
-

Name: ____________________

Date Started: ____________ Date Completed: ____________

Work Summary 2

Section 1

1. Record the numbers of the Action Papers marked "Rush." ________
2. Record the numbers of the Action Papers marked "ASAP." ________
3. Record the numbers of the Action Papers marked "Routine." ________

Section 2

4. Write the list of "To Do" items and the actions that were taken. When this section is complete, turn the Work Summary over to your instructor, who will evaluate your work and return it for your later use.

To Do	Action Taken
________	________
________	________
________	________
________	________
________	________
________	________

Section 3

5. You will receive two assessments for your work—one is based on time to complete the items and the other is based on quality of work. Your instructor will complete the Assessment portion of the Work Summary.

			Points Received
Time Required			________
	20 points	25 minutes or less	
	15 points	30 minutes	
	10 points	35 minutes	
	5 points	40 minutes	
Quality of Work			________
		Total Points	________

Name: ______________________ Date: ______________

CHAPTER 3
Medical Ethics

Chapter Outline

- Medical Ethics and the Law
- Ethics Statements of the Medical Associations
  - AMA Principles of Medical Ethics
  - American Hospital Association
  - American Association of Medical Assistants
- Social Policy Issues
  - Abortion
  - Abuse of Children, Elderly Persons, and Others at Risk
  - Allocation of Health Resources
  - In Vitro Fertilization
  - Capital Punishment
  - Clinical Investigation
  - Fetal Research Guidelines
  - Genetic Counseling and Genetic Engineering
    - Genetic Counseling
    - Genetic Engineering
  - Organ Transplantation Guidelines
  - Quality of Life
  - Terminal Illness
  - HIV Testing
  - Drug and Substance Abuse
  - Costs
  - Unnecessary Services and Worthless Services
- Computers and Ethics
  - Confidentiality and Computers
  - AMA Position on Computer Security
- The Medical Assistant's Role in Ethical Issues
  - Appropriate Patient Charges
  - Confidentiality
- Chapter Activities
  - Performance-Based Activities
  - Expanding Your Thinking

Key Vocabulary Terms

Match each word or term with its correct meaning.

_____ 1. Bioethics
_____ 2. DNR
_____ 3. Durable power of attorney
_____ 4. Genetic counseling
_____ 5. Genetic engineering
_____ 6. Genetics
_____ 7. Living will
_____ 8. Medical ethics
_____ 9. Medical law
_____ 10. Patient-Care Partnership (Patient's Bill of Rights)
_____ 11. Patient Self-Determination Act
_____ 12. Confidentiality

a. gives medical authority to one person
b. study of genes
c. extraordinary care instructions
d. basic guidelines for hospital care
e. standards set by elected officials
f. federal law on extraordinary care
g. the medical ethics of moral issues
h. advanced means of replacing genes
i. maintaining secret patient information
j. principles governing medical conduct
k. counseling related to gene disorders
l. not to prolong life through extraordinary means

Chapter Review

1. What is the difference between medical ethics and medical law?

2. Why do medical associations develop statements of ethics?

3. Every physician must take the Hippocratic Oath. Why is this oath important?